The Crossed Organization of Brains

The Crossed Organization of Brains

Edison K. Miyawaki, M.D.

Copyright © 2018 by Edison K. Miyawaki, M.D.

Library of Congress Control Number: 2018907367
ISBN: Hardcover 978-1-9845-3651-8
Softcover 978-1-9845-3650-1
eBook 978-1-9845-3649-5

All rights reserved. No part of this book may be reproduced or transmitted in any form or by any means, electronic or mechanical, including photocopying, recording, or by any information storage and retrieval system, without permission in writing from the copyright owner.

Any people depicted in stock imagery provided by Getty Images are models, and such images are being used for illustrative purposes only.
Certain stock imagery © Getty Images.

Print information available on the last page.

Rev. date: 06/21/2018

To order additional copies of this book, contact:
Xlibris
1-888-795-4274
www.Xlibris.com
Orders@Xlibris.com
781323

CONTENTS

1 Background 1
2 A Problem with Teleologies 4
3 Organization and Information 7
4 The Singular Phenomenon of Decussation 14
5 Start from Scratch 21
6 An Aside on Eyes Moving Conjugately 27
7 After the Tenth Week 32
8 "Fate" 36
9 A Note about Cartography 42
10 Point A to . . . ? 46
11 The Room 54
12 Why? 57

References 59

1

Background

The medical student's question couldn't have been more innocent or sincere. "The right brain controls the left body; the left brain, the right body. Why?"

A thoughtful answer requires a few pages.

Before we address the why, is the student's statement completely correct? If one asked a non-medical person today, "what comes to mind when I say 'right brain'?" maybe the answer would be "art," "creativity," or something aside from "control of the left body." Our student is in medical school, so she or he refers to knowledge we teach there–for example, that the cerebral cortex has to do with voluntary movement. To understand in what way the cerebral cortex and movement are related, we ask students to visualize or to draw a pyramidal tract (*tractus* in Latin refers to a drawing) starting, say, in the left frontal brain.

Axons arising from large pyramidal ("Betz") neurons in the fifth layer of the left primary motor cortex, located anterior to the central sulcus, make up part–by no means all–of the fibers of the left internal capsule. Many, not all, left internal capsular fibers eventually form the left pyramid in the medulla, and the majority of those fibers will cross the midline–they will "decussate"–in the low medulla to form a contralateral, right corticospinal tract in the spinal cord. To repeat, not all fibers of the pyramidal tract cross the midline in the low medulla, but most do. Interruptions of the tract on the left side above the decussation or on the right side below it will impair movement in the right hemibody. The pyramidal tract is an example of crossed organization in the brain. So the left brain, we conclude with some rationality, *does* control movement in the right body. Nevertheless, there are exceptions to the student's statement: some tracts in brain anatomy never cross the midline. "Control" of half of the body involves both crossed and uncrossed organizations.

What's an example of an uncrossed tract? Let's discuss just one. The vestibular system is also involved in the control of movement. We can draw a vestibulospinal tract, for example, in the right brain. (There's both a medial and a lateral vestibulospinal tract; neither crosses the midline. We will concentrate on the lateral one.) A vestibule, from the Latin, refers to some separate space, like a hotel lobby at a distance from your room. The vestibular apparatus is located in an intricately hollowed cavity in the temporal bone at a distance from the brain and brainstem. As with other afferent inputs to brain, fibers carrying information from vestibular sensory epithelia have cell bodies in a ganglion–so-called Scarpa's ganglion, which is located inside the vestibular nerve itself. Vestibular afferent fibers (from the right vestibule) innervate several vestibular nuclei in the right brainstem, but there's something unique about the lateral vestibular nucleus (of Deiter), from whence fibers of the lateral vestibulospinal tract arise. The main afferents to the right, lateral vestibular nucleus are axons from Purkinje cells of the right, paramedian vermis of cerebellum. Then a right, lateral vestibulospinal tract originates in Deiter's nucleus and descends, without decussation, in the ventrolateral spinal cord as far as lumbar levels. It's a pathway which facilitates limb extension and inhibits limb flexion on the same side of the body.

Maybe the student wasn't worried so much about what the brain controls. The real curiosity had to do with the anatomical existence of crossroads. Without comment about the control of anything, let's concede that there are crossed and uncrossed pathways in all kinds of nervous systems. Reflex action in a nerve net, like a hydra's, has nothing to do with some decussation of fibers across the midline axis of a hydra. Likewise, if I tap a patellar tendon at a human knee, a normal reflex response has to do with neural connections only on one side of the body. One needn't talk about crossed tracts at all. Vertebrate nervous systems certainly have decussations, but contemporary studies of literally all the connections among the 300-odd neurons of *C. elegans* find that some projections cross the midline, some don't, but decussations occur even in that humble, invertebrate worm.

If we remain in medical school, we memorize the pathways relevant to the practice of human neurology. We can commit to knowing the stolid facts—where specifically a pathway crosses the midline and which pathways never cross. Then, to borrow Ramon y Cajal's lovely phrase, maybe we can think at long last about "the texture of the nervous system"—in effect, truly how it is woven, rather than ask why it is woven as it is.

All the same, the medical student's question is hard to avoid for anyone interested in the structure of brains. A teacher worth the title should venture some kind of answer.

2

A Problem with Teleologies

In front of me, I have three papers which I have read and reread in preparing for this monograph. Over the next three chapters, in reverse chronological order of their publication dates, I'll discuss the arguments I found most interesting in each. All the articles have to do with what has been called the teleology of decussation. A word to the wise will suffice as we start: the telos–literally, the end–isn't known, because we haven't arrived there yet. When one thinks teleologically, one guesses about the final, definitive purpose of something. But one really doesn't know.

The strangest of the papers, by Kinsbourne from 2013, wrestles with an idea which he advanced first in the 1970's, although similar notions had been discussed as early as the 1820's. A major structural difference between a crayfish (an invertebrate) and a vertebrate has to do with where the neuraxis is located in relationship to the digestive tract. A cephalic swelling that we identify as the invertebrate brain, just like the vertebrate brain, lies dorsal to the oropharnyx and digestive tract, but the neuraxis (read: the rest of the contiguous nervous system) is ventral to the digestive tract in invertebrates.

We should pause a moment to visualize the schema fully. If I'm a crayfish, my brain is above and behind my mouth just as my human brain is, but my spinal cord passes to the front of me, anterior/ventral to my esophagus, stomach, and the rest of my bowel. But I am human–what follows applies to sharks and other chordates as well as all vertebrates—, so: my brain, spinal cord, and my spine (the notochord in a chordate) are all posterior/dorsal to my gut.

On the other hand, an obvious similarity between crayfish and humans is bilateral symmetry along the body's length. Evolutionists have long speculated about an "ur"-bilaterian creature whose axial symmetry anticipates all subsequent invertebrate, chordate, and vertebral body plans. Interspecies conservation of genes between vertebrates and invertebrates (like homeotic HOX genes in embryonic development) argues for the possibility of such a primordial common ancestor. At some point in the transition to the vertebrate nervous system and body, Kinsbourne maintains, maybe the brain stayed in one place, but the body twisted 180 degrees so that the brain, spinal cord, and spine together became dorsal to the gut.

At the risk of seeming obtuse, if the body twists relative to the head, yes, crossing of axons in a neuraxis would occur, but what about the esophagus: does it twist as well? Kinsbourne doesn't talk about the fate of the esophagus. Instead, he asks us to consider the location of the typical invertebrate heart. It lies dorsally, and blood gets pumped to the belly, flows posteriorly, and returns to the heart dorsally. In a chordate or vertebrate, the heart is ventral, and blood pulsates to the dorsum, and returns to the heart via ventral, large veins. There's an invertebrate-to-vertebrate cardiovascular twist, it seems, to support Kinsbourne, but I still wonder about that esophagus. Does it untwist eventually in evolution for the survival of species, because all animals need to get food down somehow?

What seems to matter most to the author is the predictive power of his concept. He says that there should never be an organism—"no organism should come to light" are his precise words—in which the neuraxis is dorsal, but decussation is absent. He's clever, because he avoids saying that there can't be an organism with a ventral neuraxis in which decussation does occur. Worms with some decussating fibers aren't an impossibility. But the sample crossing that we mapped in drawing a pyramidal tract, among other decussating tracts in anatomy, is a necessary consequence of a momentous occurrence in evolution.

The body didn't twist in relation to a fixed brain location in space specifically for the purpose of creating decussations. Fibers crossing the midline—or not crossing—could happen for myriad reasons, but if you buy the telos of a vertebrate body plan (with an endoskeletal spine, a dorsal neuraxis, dorsal brain, a ventral heart) then nerve fibers must cross. One could speak of a *sine qua non* of vertebrate existence: if vertebrate, then decussation perforce.

The medical student's question comes to mind once more, as it will throughout these chapters: "OK, so why does the right brain have to do with left body and vice versa?" An answer, based on the first of our papers, would be: because crossing is an epiphenomenon. ("If you are a vertebrate . . . that's just the way it is" might be another way of saying the same thing.) The author talks about his "model for the evolution of decussation," but the model isn't technically about decussation at all. It's about how vertebrates look anatomically in comparison to invertebrates. Indeed there are differences between the two types of living beings, but didn't we learn as much in some distant biology class?

3

Organization and Information

Next comes a perspective from engineering and mathematics. A virtue in this second of three papers is the attention it pays to sensory information directed to the cortex. Consider the technical question the authors (bioengineer Shinbrot and neuroscientist Young, both quite mathematically inclined) pose: what are the "constraints" on getting information from one place to another? I will take some liberty in explaining why constraints should enter into consideration at all. The following vignette is mine, not the authors', but it helps me begin to understand their paper and the concepts in it.

Let's say something lightly touches the dorsum of my left hand–in the middle of the dorsum of my left hand, just below the bottom of my middle finger, not as far down as the wrist. I know rather precisely where the touch is. In fact, I could touch the very spot in question with my right forefinger if need be. How do I know that the touch didn't occur in the palm of my left hand? It's an absurd question, of course: the back of my left hand is where the information is, so to speak, not involving the palm at all.

When the touch happened, I neglected to mention that I had my left hand palm-side down, but not resting on anything. Now I flip my left hand palm-side up, and the touch happens again at exactly the same spot on the dorsum. The location of the touch in three-dimensional space has likely changed a bit. But the surface location of the stimulus on the left dorsum has not changed. A first constraint, almost too obvious to bother mentioning but important nonetheless, is that whatever pathways are involved in the perception of the light touch, the coordinates of location relate to my left hand, not some x, y, z location in extra-personal space.

We've described discrete events: 1. a touch on the dorsum of the left hand at a precise spot with the palm facing down and 2. a touch at the same spot on the dorsum with the palm facing up. If there were a map of some kind representing my hand, would there be one or two locations for the two events? If one answers "just one, on the dorsum" then how to account for the changed position of the left hand? The difference matters, because if I wanted to touch the spot on the left with my right forefinger, the task differs depending on whether my left hand is palm down or up. Does one need a different map, more three dimensional perhaps, in which the spot on the left dorsum gets two representations, one with the left hand palm-side down and another with the left hand palm-side up? Three dimensionality (any possible location of the hand in external space as the touch occurs) introduces not so much a constraint as a seemingly limitless quantity of information to be mapped somehow.

We spoke at the start about information "getting" from one place to another, so let's perform rudimentary connections between two maps. Map one–call it "actual left hand"–has a black dot on it, representing the spot of the touch, but for the sake of distinguishing dorsum from palm, we place a red dot on the flip side of Map one's surface (anywhere will do). Map two–call it "virtual left hand"–also has a black dot on it on its dorsum and likewise a red dot on the reverse, palmar side. Connect black dot with black dot and red with red (reading this chapter's paper had me playing with index cards and string; I literally did connect dots). Flip Map one 180 degrees, and there will be crossing of the strings, unless you flip Map two 180 degrees in the same direction.

The authors say that such point-to-point connectivity, when it comes to representing a three-dimensional location *on the virtual map*, is cumbersome. And it is without question, especially if you consider that connecting dots between actual and virtual maps would involve a surfeit of crossings if, for example, we tracked the progress of an ant walking across the dorsum of the hand towards the palm then down the side of a finger. Note that the crossing of strings between dots is not a decussation of fibers across the body's midline. In our vignette, the virtual map and the actual map are homolateral to each other. Pathways/strings between actual and virtual (by analogy, respectively: body map and hypothetical brain map) will crisscross, but no midline decussation occurs at all.

The authors think that an inescapable problem in representing three-dimensional sensory information is messiness and disorganization. Like a law that can't be violated without deleterious consequences, a constraint operates in the cortical representation of sensory data. It is a statute of neatness or efficiency. The telos is an unmessy, organized transfer of information from the periphery to the brain. In a modest edit of the medical student's question, how does decussation across a midline help to organize information, especially in three dimensions?

Now is a good time to review a pathway that has to do with the perception of light touch in humans, though it has been studied most carefully in other animals. Although we'll discuss the lemniscal system in particular, I'll direct attention to a structural feature that is also an aspect of another ascending tract mediating pain and temperature sensation.

The lightest touch on the dorsum, again, of the left hand is a phenomenon in and of itself that we could discuss for a while. Did hair follicles move with the touch? Did the touch involve some slight movement across the skin or just pressure in one place? Did the touch involve heat or cold? What is "touch"? To simplify, let's talk about a mechanical activation of some tactile corpuscles in the skin there, a bit of information that finds its way to consciousness, if we become aware that our left hand has been touched.

Light-touch sensory fibers in the peripheral nervous system are said to be generously myelinated with swift conduction times, but some investigators talk about a mix of degrees of myelination in sensory nerves mediating light touch. The cell bodies of the axons in question are located in a dorsal root ganglion, which lies in close proximity to the dorsal side of the spinal cord. (We'll concentrate on the left cervical cord, because the information comes from the dorsum of the left hand.) From the dorsal root ganglion, without a synapse, fibers will enter the cord heading into a fasciculus (a bundle) in the dorsal column of the cord. There's little argument about the amount of myelin in a dorsal column: the fascicles there are thickly myelinated.

We are now in the cuneate fasciculus—the column of Burdach, if you learn anatomy in Europe—in the dorsolateral left spinal cord. More specifically, there has been a transformation of mechanical activation into an electrical signal, and the signal (call it just one action potential, for the sake of simplicity) travels along a myelinated axon in the cuneate fasciculus. A synapse will occur in the cuneate nucleus, located rostrally, at the cervicomedullary junction. I should call it by its proper name: it is the medial cuneate nucleus, because there's also a lateral (accessory) cuneate nucleus, which is associated with a different ascending tract to cerebellum rather than cerebrum.

Before the synapse in the medial cuneate nucleus occurs, where's the spot on the dorsum of the left hand represented?

We say that there is somatotopic organization at all levels of the lemniscal system, as is true for other somatic sensory pathways. Sensory information from the leg ascends in the dorsomedial cord in the gracile fasciculus, from the arm and hand dorsolaterally in the cuneate fasciculus; we refer to such parcellation as somatotopic. But a sense of anatomical order suggested by the word "somatotopy" needs to be adjusted when we think about how the hand is represented in the medial cuneate nucleus. In a portion of that nucleus called the pars rotunda, the hand's map is deconstructed and rearranged.

If, at this very moment, I look at the back of my left hand, I see, moving proximal to distal: my wrist, my dorsum, then my knuckled, wrinkled fingers. If I look at a coronal section of the pars rotunda in the medial cuneate nucleus, the representation of the hand, going dorsal to ventral, is: dorsum of hand, palm, dorsal fingertips, palmar fingertips—to simplify: back, front, back, front, with dorsum and palm *above* the fingers (Florence et al., 1989).

Maybe the above is knowledge that only an anatomist could love. The point is: before decussation across the midline (we'll trace it in a moment), there's a routing of connections to a curious-looking map of the hand in the medial cuneate nucleus. To create such a map likely necessitates crossings of connections just as in the flip of Map one relative to Map two that we described earlier.

Let's now track the course of the second-order neuron in the lemniscal system. As is also true in the anterolateral sensory pathway, a second-order neuron, not the first-order neuron, will cross the midline. From the medial cuneate nucleus, after a synapse, second-order axons cross from the left side to a medial, vertically oriented tract, the right medial lemniscus. The fibers arch through the central medulla on both sides (the internal arcuate fibers, which cross the midline). In the medial lemniscus, now in the right brainstem, representation of the left arm and hand is dorsal to that of the leg and foot. All the fibers, literally in a ribbon (a lemniscus), will wind their way rostrally towards the ventroposterior nuclear group of the right thalamus, then to right parietal cortex. The decussation of leminscal fibers happens a little higher (a bit more rostrally) than the decussation of the pyramidal tracts in the motor system.

The basic pathway that we have sketched invites mathematical considerations, according to our authors. The math involves the likelihood of wiring errors if the number of elements connected to each other is large and if the number of turns to be negotiated is also large. The authors say that a fully decussated arrangement across the midline of just 1,000 connections between brain and body maps, as opposed to an undecussated arrangement, reduces the probability of wiring error by at least an order of magnitude.

They offer a computer simulation (first using brain and body maps with 1,000 nodes each without decussation) to demonstrate that when you introduce a very small error factor each time over 100,000 iterations, then somatotopic correlation–the connections–between brain and body maps go very awry (and they stay that way) after just 10,000 trials. But in a decussated arrangement, rather few non-somatotopic connections ever arise at any point in the simulation, well past the 10,000 mark by an order of magnitude. Since miswiring in neurobiology is inherently disadvantageous and because error in complex systems is inescapable, there "should be an evolutionary drive toward decussated networks"—"should be," because the best way to transfer information is to keep it organized and as error free as possible.

I'll draw an analogy to a hypothetical city divided by a river that runs east to west. I'm interested to get from point A in the southwest of the city to point B northeast. My plan is to take a major subway line across the river. Its station can be found at the center of the city on the southern bank of the river. Crossing at that one place reduces the possibility of my getting lost in getting from south to north.

There's an oddity to this urban landscape. Landmarks in the southwest and northeast are reduplicated, as if there were two Eiffel Towers in Paris. Indeed the whole northern city looks similar to the southern city. Clearly, I've made a mistake. Maybe I turned my map upside down at the subway station, because tourists get confused easily.

Or: something could have happened to southern information at the point of transfer across the river.

Fibers decussate after synapsing in the medial caudate nucleus. In that nucleus, the map of the hand already looks different than my left hand, and we know very well that the homuncular representations in thalamus and sensory cortex exaggerate—they even reduplicate—some parts of the body while maintaining a semblance of somatotopy.

We simply can't talk about a single homuncular representation anywhere in the subsequent course of the lemniscal pathway after its decussation. Sensory cortical maps, taking just Brodmann's areas 3a (at the bottom of the central sulcus), 3b (caudal bank of central sulcus), 1 (a large part of the postcentral gyrus, visible on the lateral surface), and 2 (caudal to 1, but without extension to the medial surface of the brain), reduplicate homuncular representations. The multiple homunculi lie in a columnar arrangement next to each other in Brodmann's areas 3a, 3b, 1, and 2.

Then there's the anterolateral system, which we've not traced in detail, except to notice that second-order neurons also cross the midline in that distinct ascending system. Second-order fibers arise after synapsing in the substantia gelatinosa to cross segmentally in the cord in anterior white commissures at many levels. After crossing, the anterolateral system ascends on the opposite side towards the thalamus and cortex. The parsimony afforded by decussation, i.e., a reduced error rate, might still apply if we think about the pathway mediating pain and temperature, but why so many crossings?

The interest in Shinbrot and Young's paper is its claim that decussation is anything but a random biological phenomenon. It occurred for the limitation of wrong connections. It's a lovely argument, but the anatomy is even more beautiful and humbling than the authors' mathematics.

4

The Singular Phenomenon of Decussation

The title of this chapter is a phrase of Cajal's. The third of our papers owes much to his cogitation on the incomplete crossing of fibers in the visual system—which we will discuss in what follows. But, in their first pages, the authors (Vulliemoz, Raineteau, and Jabaudon) teach me a fact which I'll accept at face value; it's worth a moment's consideration: in non-mammalian vertebrates, tracts that originate in the brainstem control *most* motor functions. By "most," they refer to practicalities such as control of muscular tone, of posture, and the maintenance of balance of an entire body. Tracts arising in the brainstem are numerous, but a short list would include: reticulospinal, tectospinal, vestibulospinal, and rubrospinal. Which of these cross the midline?

Let me phrase the question differently. Would you expect all of them *not* to cross the midline? We have introduced the lateral vestibulospinal tract arising from Deiter's lateral vestibular nucleus, and we said that it facilitates extensor tone on the same side of the body without decussation across the midline. It would make teaching and memorization so much easier if we could say, "if a descending motor tract arises in the brainstem, then it's an uncrossed tract." The statement isn't true, unfortunately, but I find it interesting that, depending on where a brainstem motor tract originates, some cross the midline and others don't.

Officially to answer the question, then, the tectospinal and rubrospinal tracts (arising from the superior colliculus and red nucleus, respectively) cross the midline, whereas the reticulospinal and vestibulospinal tracts (arising from pontine and medullary portions of the reticular formation and medullary vestibular nuclei, respectively) do not. Someone will object that reticulospinal fibers sometimes do cross the midline at a lower point, maybe in the low medulla or in the spinal cord. That person, even if technically correct, misses the singularity that Cajal observes about decussations.

They are singularly obvious. It doesn't take effort to see the decussation of the pyramids at the cervicomedullary junction: it effaces the anterior median fissure on the ventral surface. Intraaxially, we can see decussating internal arcuate fibers in the transition from the medial caudate or gracile nuclei to the medial lemnisci on either side. Likewise, tectospinal tracts manifestly cross in a dorsal tegmental decussation in midbrain. And rubrospinal tracts cross in a ventral tegmental decussation in the midbrain. At the level of the third nerve nuclear complex (visualize a canonical axial microphotograph of a midbrain, with obvious red nuclei and the shark tooth appearance of nucleus of cranial nerve III in the middle), a lot of midline crossing happens near and around those red nuclei. Consider, as an additional example, the decussation of the superior cerebellar peduncles just caudal to the level just mentioned. Decussation simply isn't subtle; it's a plain phenomenon. Crossings across the midline vexed Cajal, because their functional benefit to an organism struck him as "obscure."

So, in non-mammalian vertebrates, brainstem pathways control most motor functions. What's to be done after "most" control has been achieved? The authors talk about exceptional motor capacities that supervene once most motor control has been accomplished. As the telencephalon develops in size and complexity from non-mammal to the human mammal, is decussation necessary for increasingly exceptional capacities? The authors say yes.

*

Let's consider a particularly obvious chiasm in anatomy.

About 165 years before Cajal, Isaac Newton anatomized binocular vision. Here is query 15 from Book Three of his *Opticks* (note that this third part of the book is a series of questions, rather than the "propositions" one finds elsewhere in the work): "Are not the Species of Objects seen with both Eyes united where the optick Nerves meet before they come into the Brain, the Fibres on the right side of both Nerves uniting there, and after union going thence into the Brain in the Nerve [what we would now call the tract] which is on the right side of the Head . . . [?] . . . For the optick Nerves of such Animals as look the same way with both Eyes (as of Men, Dogs, Sheep, Oxen, &c) meet before they come into the Brain, but the optick Nerves of such Animals as do not look the same way with both Eyes (as of Fishes, and of the Chameleon) do not meet, if I am rightly inform'd."

In response to Sir Isaac, who is neuroanatomically correct about the human optic chiasm, I'll digress briefly.

Since my own introductory anatomy days in school, I've wondered whether animals who have eyes on the sides of their heads, who seem to look laterally rather than in a forward direction, have optic chiasms or visual pathway decussations. Then, one day–in one of those scholarly fishing expeditions that can occupy a person for a whole afternoon or more–I found a paper entitled "Stereopsis in Toads." Like chameleons, toads have quite laterally displaced eyes, but unlike chameleons, to make matters apparently worse for toads, toads' eyes barely move in their sockets. Yet toads achieve depth perception (stereopsis); they have optic chiasms; and–here's a remarkable observation–toads have a visual field of almost 360 degrees, due to binocular overlap that is both in front of and, importantly, *above* the eyes. I'll spare the reader comments about the visually-guided accuracy of a toad's tongue dart for food in three-dimensional space. The take-home from my digression is, simply, that "Animals as do not look the same way with both Eyes" nevertheless have chiasms. Newton was slightly misinformed.

Vulliemoz, Raineteau, and Jabaudon invoke Cajal's conjecture (from 1898) that, in the course of evolution, the more fibers cross in an optic chiasm the *less* likely one would observe decussating motor fibers. Does the inverse relationship make sense? A visual datum in left external space transmits to the right brain of a vertebrate without limbs. Let's say that the crossing is absolutely complete: all ganglion cell axons from the left retina transmit to the right brain. Then (so runs the conjecture) descending, uncrossed motor pathways in the right brain drive movement in the right hemibody—for example, the right side contracts to evade or extends to approach the datum in left external space. There's no need for a decussating motor pathway.

To consider a more exceptional task under visual guidance, we need to know about a visual pathway that doesn't completely cross.

I like to start with ganglion cells in the retina, because we are discussing a fiber tract. The outgoing axons in question belong to retinal ganglion cells. Not all ganglion cells connect to other retinal cells the same way. At the fovea (or "macula," but I like the word fovea), one cone connects to one bipolar cell then to one retinal ganglion cell. Elsewhere, the connection is less one to one. For the retina as a whole, the ratio of all light receptors (cones and rods) to ganglion cells is estimated to be 125:1.

In the periphery of the retina, as opposed to the fovea, more cones and rods connect to more bipolar cells, which connect to the relatively parsimonious number of ganglion cells. The fovea, just to state what's well known, is responsible for our acutest vision. And in the fovea, retinal ganglion axons in its nasal half are destined to cross the midline, those in the temporal half will not. The naso-temporal division is not always clear in other species, but in primates and humans, it's very sharp.

Temporal retinal and foveal fibers that do not cross terminate in various locations, among them the pretectal nuclei, the superior colliculus, and even the suprachiasmatic nucleus in hypothalamus, in addition to the lateral geniculate nucleus, all on the same side. Fibers that do cross—only those nasal to the nasotemporal division of the whole retina and its fovea—will terminate in the contralateral superior colliculus and lateral geniculate nucleus, not to the other locations just mentioned.

Whether crossing in the visual pathway is complete or partial, our authors tell us, depends on the existence of binocular vision—or, stereopsis. In brief, they offer us two claims to consider. First, partial crossing is necessary for stereopsis. Second, stereopsis is so necessary for exceptional motor acts that the pathways responsible for those acts (like the corticospinal tract) will decussate in relationship to the development of stereopsis. Though I don't doubt that binocular vision is a useful attribute for tasks performed under visual guidance, I have a problem with the second claim, based on the anatomy that supports the first. I also hear the medical student quizzing me with exasperation: "The corticospinal tract crosses, because the visual pathway partially crosses, because we're visual animals? Really, that's what you've got?"

The lateral geniculate nucleus (also known as the lateral geniculate body) is the terminus of the optic tract. One of my teachers had this to say about binocular vision and that nucleus (from a book entitled *Eye, Brain, and Vision*): "The lateral geniculate body represents the first opportunity for information from the two eyes to come together at the level of a single cell. But it seems that the opportunity there is missed: the two sets of input are consigned to separate sets of layers, with little or no opportunity to combine. As we would expect from this segregation, a geniculate cell responds to one eye and not at all to the other" (Hubel, 1995).

The opportunity is missed rather completely, in fact. Among the six cellular layers of the lateral geniculate nucleus, any one layer or any cell in that one layer deals either with left or right eye information, despite the fact that fibers from both eyes converge in the lateral geniculate nucleus. For stereopsis to happen, information kept so very discrete must merge somewhere. Question: where? My teacher's answer is: the cerebral cortex and at no point prior to it. The comment stuns by its simplicity.

I have a task in mind as I describe the visual pathway and its relationship to motor control. I'm threading a needle. Certainly it's a task under visual guidance. The high likelihood is that I perform this act in a well-lit place, and odds are that the needle and thread are oriented toward my foveae. I want to maximize the likelihood of success on my first attempt. I've already moistened the thread, which I hold between my right thumb and forefinger; the eye of the needle faces my eyes, which point inwardly in slight accommodation. The needle is fixed in space, more or less (due to my little tremor), with my left forefinger and thumb. Like some often do, I close one eye, because it seems I see better with one eye than the other. In my case, I close my left eye just for a moment. I thread the needle. Was stereopsis involved?

At least both motor cortices—whatever controls movement in both my hands—must be engaged in this task, which requires that I know where objects are in space and at what relative depth. One surmises that stereopsis must be involved, with activity in visual cortex.

All of a sudden, questions come to mind. Which visual cortex? Both of them? When I close my left eye to spot the eye of the needle keenly, don't I temporarily yield binocularity? But monocular information from my right eye reaches both cortices—nasal right retinal information heads to left cortex by crossing the midline; temporal right retinal information heads to right cortex without crossing. We've traced the pathway as far as the lateral geniculate nucleus, which only has cells specific to right or left eye. Truly binocular cells are a cortical matter, as my teacher said. For a fine motor skill, performed just in front of my midline (in front of my nose, actually), I'd say that a whole lot of my cortex—motoric and visual—is active, on both sides. Stereopsis simply invites consideration of how both cortices can be involved in trivial needle threading.

I can't wholly agree with the authors when they suggest that visual wiring influenced the development of a decussating corticospinal tract. They rephrase Cajal's conjecture, and of course it's an affront to disagree with a Cajal. But what does "influence" mean? It's a squishy verb.

We can say instead that there must be a lot of midline crossing in motor and visual systems alike for information to get where it needs to go in the task of needle threading. Both cerebral cortices are likely involved, and the hemispheres must engage each other—they must communicate in real time—somehow.

*

The remainder of the third paper in our series has to do with syndromes in which decussations are absent, with a variety of clinical consequences. One of the syndromes, first described in the late 1960's, will be a topic in a later chapter. For now, we're not done discussing a basic anatomy of crossings, but we're in a position to summarize what all three papers have taught us so far.

One doubts that the fabled missing link will be found, the first or ur-vertebrate whose body twists up to 180 degrees relative to the brain. Vertebrate and chordate body plans inescapably have dorsal neuraxes and endoskeletons, but it's a misstatement to say that crossing doesn't happen in invertebrates. In a vertebrate, however, crossing results in a bicameral arrangement in which one half of the brain represents or deals with the opposite half of space.

Depicting space in three dimensions on a cortical map—the main subject matter of the second paper of the three I chose—is a non-trivial information problem prone to error, and maybe midline decussation organizes data.

A question as benign as "forget decussations for a moment, why are there even *tracts* in anatomy?" begins to resemble the medical student's original question in kind. Why "tracts" at all? A tract keeps like fibers together in discrete boulevards; similarly, decussation allows like fibers to achieve their analogous positions on cortical maps with less likelihood of losing their way. The answer to queries about tracts and decussations is: less error, to which biology and life is prone.

Then, based on a conjecture by Cajal, the authors of the third paper contemplate actions performed by the nervous system when "most" motor control has been achieved. We've considered a task requiring bimanual dexterity performed right in front of eyes pointing forward, and we infer that halves of the brain are communicating to accomplish the threading of a needle.

Crossing is manifest in brain anatomy. A non-mundane question arises because of that singular phenomenon. It's a question in two parts. We basically discuss sidedness—right side of brain, left side of the world, etc. When do sides happen in the brain? Then: how do sides communicate?

We need more anatomy, because we haven't at all exhausted how much crossing there is.

5

Start from Scratch

If there's one course in medical school, or part of a course, that I'd take again from scratch, it would be embryology. Dusting off my copy of Langman's *Medical Embryology*, which was in its fourth edition in the 1980's, I turn to the last chapter, on the central nervous system. (It seems that the nervous system occupies the backside of all general medical textbooks.) Way back when, by the time I got to Langman's chapter 20, the embryology final exam was imminent, my exhaustion complete, and the intellect dissipated. But it's the neuro-development part of the course I'd retake today. I read on the chapter's first page that a flattish thickening of ectoderm, called a neural plate, appears early in the third gestational week in humans, and that closure of the cranial neuropore occurs around day 25.

Fast forward from a horrid first year of school to the second year of neurology training, during months at a place called TCH, for *The* Children's Hospital, as opposed to a children's hospital. There, a teacher of sphinx-like demeanor taught that a given brain malformation may not have its onset after a developmental event is completed. The statement—in fact, it was an end-stop pronouncement that left silence in its wake—strikes me as a riddle to this day. Here's a variation of the riddle for present purposes: when do right and left connect in brains? We ask, not only because we want to know when connections start, but also when they might go astray.

Upon closure of the cranial neuropore, in what is otherwise called "induction" on the dorsal side of the embryo (there's yet another synonym: dorsal induction is also known as primary neurulation), is *that* when right and left connect?

Take out another trusty index card (this time it's my model of a neural plate). Indulge me by drawing a thick line with a Sharpie right down the middle of the card lengthwise. We'll call this line the ventral extent of tube. Appose the left and right side of the card, with the Sharpie line on the inside of the tube. Apply tape to the seam along the whole length. The tape marks the dorsal side.

I've joined right and left sides of the card together, but the only demarcations are the Sharpie line and the dorsal seam. We have modeled dorsal induction.

To make my index-card exercise a bit more rigorous, I head to a website like "Online Mendelian Inheritance in Man" (I try GeneCards and EntrezGene as well). I enter "dorsal neural tube induction." Like a jackpot on the computer screen, there's immediately more genetics in front of me than I can know at a glance. There are names like wingless, snail family transcriptional repressor (slug), bone morphogenetic protein (BMP), paired box (PAX), sonic hedgehog (SHH), many more. In the aggregate, the talk is about dorsal vs. ventral genetic expression, not right vs. left. For example, wingless proteins (Wnt) are found more on the dorsal side of the neural tube; sonic hedgehog (the protein) concentrates ventrally. The molecular mechanisms of induction are the stuff of current embryology courses, as students today know all too well.

The great sphinx of TCH would say that once dorsal induction and closure of the cranial neuropore occurs, you can't *not* have a brain, as in cases of craniorachischisis totalis or anencephaly. Unanswered, however, is the matter of right and left sides and the connections between the two. The cranial neuropore was once an open end to the neural tube; it closes by apposition of its sides as guided by multiple genes and their proteins. Do interhemispheric connections happen at that time? The sphinx shrugs in response. "At this time, there are no hemispheres," I hear him in my ear.

Dorsal induction happens at approximately three to four weeks' gestation. Ventral induction happens at approximately five-to-six weeks' gestation. To get as efficiently as possible to our interest at five-to-six weeks, look back a few sentences to note the word "ventral" (as in ventral neural tube) associated with sonic hedgehog, the protein. Its gene, SHH, is located on chromosome seven; its expression happens along the ventral neural tube in the midline.

Now, consider three observations together: 1. Ventral induction, when complete after the sixth week, results in *paired* cerebral hemispheres; the corpus callosum across hemispheres myelinates (appears) later; 2. There can't be onset of holoprosencephaly after the fifth or sixth week, but when it occurs, the most severe cases are characterized by an undivided cortical mantle, a midline single ventricle, no olfactory bulbs or tracts, sometimes a single optic nerve to a cyclopean eye, typically no corpus callosum, and cortical histology that looks like hippocampal archicortex; 3. A spectrum of SHH mutations causes holoprosencephaly with diverse phenotypes, not all of them affecting the brain to the severest extent just mentioned.

After five-to-six weeks' gestation and after successful ventral induction, then and only then can one discuss hemispheric division under the influence of SHH (that gene, at very least). And there can't yet be any meaningful mention of neuronal connections, because myelination of axons will occur in a sequence that extends in time well past the sixth week even into young adulthood.

Actually, a first observation about connectivity in the early fetal brain might be "there's no myelin"—so, essentially, no connections. Instead, we have a TCH mantra pertinent to the first month and a half of existence. CLOSE, first (closure of the cranial neuropore); DIVIDE, second (into cerebral hemispheres); PROLIFERATE, last (neurons begin to proliferate and to migrate no earlier than at eight weeks' gestation). There's a hint of irony in all the above: you've divided left from right with no connection between what you've divided; in the first weeks of gestation, wiring isn't hard-wired.

By the way, when ventral induction occurs, the rudimentary brain doesn't only divide along the long axis. There's division in all axes: x, y, and z. Dividing top from bottom in a simplified brain sphere, we can visualize a basal (ventral/motor) versus an alar (dorsal/sensory) hemisphere. The demarcation (call it the x axis) is the sulcus limitans of Wilhelm His, Senior (his son, also an academic physician, described the heart's bundle of His); the sulcus limitans is particularly obvious in the spinal cord and the medulla oblongata. The y axis is the horizontal midline. On either side of the y axis, just now beginning to expand into z-axis space, we have the nascent hemispheres.

Paired, lateral hemispheres are the interest here. There's an ontogeny of connections between the two sides which we can review, mainly to note how much of a work-in-progress it is getting hemispheres to wire. The decussating tracts mentioned in our earlier chapters are only a small part of the crossed organization of brains.

*

Like an editor fussy about diction, the medical student groans at the word "ontogeny" and begrudgingly looks up a definition, "the course of development of an individual organism." Given that a different book, much longer than a monograph, could be written about what we now know about fetal and post-birth human myelination, a brief ontogenic review can only highlight moments in a sequence that most of us have negotiated successfully. We're interested to describe when midline connections happen and where they happen, in embryologic time.

Back to our index card. As we left it, we just had a tube with a ventral Sharpie line and a dorsal seam, nothing more. To visualize ventral induction in the fifth-to-sixth week, pinch the tube on its "cranial" end, then look down the tube's long axis. Look towards the rostral pinch. (If you insist, you can try push up just from the ventral side, in deference to "ventral induction," but just pinching one end works.)

Use your imagination, and think that you are looking through a midline ventricle (in my mind, I think the third ventricle) into the start of two lateral ventricles. The ventral Sharpie line and the dorsal seam meet in the middle where you are pinching. In this crude model, where the lines converge—at the pinch—marks the lamina terminalis in anatomy, the rostral extent of the third ventricle.

I stare down the length of the dorsal seam. My Sharpie line looks like it returns back to me ventrally, towards the center of my gaze. We can map the locations of crossings which first appear in the tenth gestational week, though, at week ten, many appear as mere shadows or premonitions compared to their mature forms.

A caveat: in terms of an axial level, we'll begin at the start of the third ventricle, so we won't comment on two interesting, more caudal crossings, the trochlear decussation and the medial longitudinal fasciculus. Those are topics for the next chapter.

The following six names may not all be familiar; I'll help with crib notes next to the names. Each of them cross the midline. Beginning dorsally, they are:

1. The posterior commissure (Think about the pupillary light reflex: how does light presented to one pupil get transferred, as information, to the other side?).
2. The habenular commissure. (From my Latin dictionary: habenula, diminutive of habena, "that by which a thing is held," like a horse rider's rein, a strap. The habenula and the pineal gland are very close to each other: how does light influence sleep?)

We move more ventrally:

3. Corpus callosum, literally the "hard body," is anterior to the lamina terminalis. It's utterly rudimentary, hardly hard, at ten weeks.
4. The hippocampal or fornical commissure, which may appear a bit later than ten weeks (fourteen weeks, according to anatomist Nieuwenhuys, 2008).
5. The anterior commissure. I'll comment on it in a moment.
6. The optic chiasm, whose myelination continues well into the seventh gestational month.

Of these six, the anterior commissure, which connects olfactory areas of the nascent cortices and the amygdalae on either side, is the first to appear. Next come the habenular and posterior commissures. The oldest tissues connect first (think: olfactory areas, habenulae, hippocampal formations). The new cortices (think: via corpus callosum) connect later.

Enlisting the hint about a posterior commissure connecting side to side in a visual pathway that has to do with external space, do these six commissures interconnect a divided brain, body, and map of the external world? There are two ways to answer. First, a too-simplistic response: yes, because sides meet. Alternatively, we might obsess over the word commissure (literally, a "commitment"–which is rather different than an accomplished connection–not a *fait accompli*, in other words).

Based on anatomy in the midline third ventricle at ten weeks' gestation, phylogenetically old brain starts to connect to with old brain on the other side, like aged collegiate alumni who "reconnect" at a dreary reunion. Someone will complain that I haven't defined old versus new brain anatomically, and that's quite correct, perhaps unforgivable. But if you want an example of a really old strap of neural tissue, the habenula is an archetype, a better example than even amygdala or hippocampus. The habenular commissure connects very old side its kindred on the other side.

*

The clock of life now reads ten weeks' gestation. Notice at this moment, there's no representation of the body, really. We have no medial lemniscus, no internal capsule, no pyramidal tract, no decussation of pyramids, and not even much of an optic chiasm.

So, when do right body and left brain and vice versa enter into their fixed and irreversible commitment to each other?

6

An Aside on Eyes Moving Conjugately

Some poor soul, a mature adult, suffers an infarction in the right hemisphere. The left body is weak, arm weaker than leg. The eyes look together, conjugately, to the right; the head turns to the right as well.

Looking away from hemiparesis (towards the lesion) in a case of cortical infarction was the subject of a 19th-century thesis by a Genevan named Jean-Louis Prévost, based on his clinical experience in Paris. He reported 51 cases. His Parisian mentor, Alfred Vulpian, gave him the idea to study the phenomenon.

Depending on the size and location of the responsible lesion in the hemisphere, deviation of the eyes can last days to weeks, but it isn't permanent. Acutely, if well enough to follow instructions, the patient would be able to look up and down when asked to do so, with both eyes moving together. But the eyes still deviate conjugately to the right in the horizontal plane.

This chapter addresses two issues having to do with eyes.

Here's the first of the two: why do eye abduction and contralateral eye adduction (and vice versa) happen together in the first place? Many medical students can't wait to blurt out the words "medial longitudinal fasciculus (or the letters M, L, and F)." Not to be harsh, but that's not an answer. The medial longitudinal fasciculus (MLF) is just a name.

It's true that the MLF contains a decussating connection between an abducens nucleus on one side and that part of the oculomotor nucleus that controls the medial rectus on the opposite side. (One adds quickly that the MLF contains much else. In fact, the majority of its fibers originate in vestibular nuclei, *not* the abducens nucleus.) It's also true that in the absence of an MLF, or if it were damaged in some way, the conjugate deviation we've described in the case of a right hemisphere stroke might differ. The MLF pertains to our discussion, absolutely.

But to answer the first of our two questions, we're on firmer ground with a less sophisticated answer, which smacks of teleology (not always good), but it is simple and not simplistic (usually good): "Assuming we aren't blind in one eye, for us to be able to move our eyes in the horizontal plane, one eye has to abduct *as* the other adducts." For good measure, we can mention equal innervation of abductor and adductor, because without it (per Ewald Hering's law of equal innervation), we run the chance of double vision with any horizontal saccade. Of note, we're not just talking about voluntary saccades towards objects in the periphery.

If my head subtly moves from side to side, to keep an object in front of me on my retinae (foveae), the eyes must move conjugately in the horizontal plane, in a direction opposite to the head movement. Prévost's observation that the head as well as the eyes turn to the side of the lesion (he says so in the title of his thesis, *"De la déviation conjugee des yeux et de la rotation de la tete dans certain cas d'hemiplegie"*) becomes a nuance of interest. Eyes (*des yeux*) rivet to the right; the patient literally rotates the head/*la tete* in that same direction, as if willfully gazing away from her or his paralysis. But it's not a willed act.

I should make an important distinction regarding "gaze." There are countless gazes, as artists know (Picasso acknowledged a native Andalusian *mirada fuerte*—"strong gazing"—as a birthright important to his art).

A neurologist distinguishes between a visually evoked movement of eyes with long latency, on the order of 100 milliseconds, and very short latency eye movements which transpire more quickly by a factor of ten, or roughly 10 milliseconds. Short latency is necessary to make the kinds of vertical, torsional, and horizontal compensations required when the head subtly moves in all planes when walking, running, etc. Short-latency eye movements have to do with the vestibulo-ocular reflex, a neural matrix of brainstem connections. Long-latency gaze, including Andalusian strong gazing, involves more of the entire brain.

We ended our last chapter curious about timing, when one side of brain definitively links to the other side of the body. In the case of the MLF, we're awfully close to definitiveness: two nuclei on opposite sides connect to each other; midline crossing happens (must happen); and the structure myelinates early.

The MLF is phylogenetically ancient, and "in ontogenesis it stands out very clearly on account of its early myelination." (That's Brodal from 1981; I quote the father, not the son. Both were anatomists.) We've discussed commissures whose primordial forms can be seen at 10 weeks' gestation. The MLF appears even earlier, at the end of the first gestational month. In many vertebrates, the MLF is the very first white-matter tract to appear in ontogeny. At full-term birth in humans, there's a short list of structures whose myelination is visible in a gross dissection. On that list are: MLF, cranial nerves, the optic chiasm and tracts (but not the optic radiations), and some other structures whose myelination is not quite as clear as the others.

*

With respect to vertical conjugate movements of eyes, here is the second of two issues in this chapter, phrased again as a question: why do eye elevation and contralateral eye extorsion happen together in the first place? I hear the medical student in a state of consternation: "what in the world *is* 'extorsion,' as opposed to the criminal act of extortion?" Issue two in this chapter is completely analogous to issue one, but we refer now to vertical rather than horizontal movement.

The general subject is why individual ocular muscles are "yoked" in the first place. Assuming we aren't blind in one eye, for us to be able to move our eyes in the vertical plane, one eye has to elevate *as* the other extorts. For good measure, we can mention equal innervation of muscles which elevate and extort, because without it (per Ewald Hering's law of equal innervation), we run the chance of double vision with any vertical saccade. Decussation is involved in the yoking of muscles; indeed, decussation has to be involved.

Regarding extorsion as opposed to extortion as opposed to elevation, look up and to your left. Your right eye extorts as your left eye elevates. Now look down and to your right. Your right eye depresses as your left eye intorts.

We've mentioned short and long latencies in generating conjugate eye movements. In the case of quick vertical compensations, we should think about a rostral part of the MLF, high up in the midbrain, at the level of the upper pole of the red nucleus. Dorsal to the red nuclei at their very tips are nuclei of the rostral interstitial MLF.

Let's orient ourselves in the midbrain for a moment. Superior colliculus is above the inferior colliculus, check. Third nerve nucleus, including its various subnuclei, is above the trochlear nucleus, the latter roughly at the level of the inferior colliculus, check. The nuclei of the rostral interstitial MLF sits just above the upper pole of the red nucleus in the high midbrain. OK, you kindly say, I'll take your word for it.

Wait, there are subnuclei of the third nerve nucleus? Yes. There are subnuclei specific to the extraocular muscles controlled by the third cranial nerve. Those muscles are the inferior oblique, the inferior rectus, the superior rectus, and the medial rectus. In terms of vertical movement of eyes, there's something unique about fibers emanating from the subnucleus associated with the superior rectus. There's also something unique about the fibers emanating from the cranial nerve nucleus of the trochlear nerve, the fourth cranial nerve. What's the uniqueness?

The word "decussation" comes to mind.

They say, whoever "they" are, that only one cranial nerve has its nucleus on the side opposite where the muscle it innervates (textbook answer: a left trochlear nucleus gives rise to the right trochlear nerve, which innervates the right superior oblique). The trochlear midline crossing happens in the anterior medullary velum, which is a veil of tissue that stretches between the two superior cerebellar peduncles on the dorsal side of midbrain. Likewise, right trochlear nucleus innervates left superior oblique. The trochlear decussation is present at ten weeks' gestation in humans.

The trochlear nucleus has a partner in decussation. What we generically teach about the curiosity of the fourth cranial nerve sniffs of misstatement.

Fibers of the superior rectus subnucleus of cranial nerve III *also cross the midline*. The left subnucleus of cranial nerve III gives rise to fibers that innervate the right superior rectus muscle.

There's an elegance in the above informational overload. There's no other word for it: elegance.

Consider that a quick vertical (upward) corrective saccade is necessary, because in a run we take one random day, with one footfall, there's a pothole we didn't expect. It's an irregular pothole. A foot gets caught in an oblique way, casting us in an oblique direction, but, mercifully, we don't fall. The run continues to our satisfaction, without injury.

As foot meets pothole, I envision events having occurred within just a few milliseconds: unilateral firing of the rostral interstitial nucleus of the MLF, say, on the left, then immediate activation of the following, all on the same side of the midline (on the left): subnuclei of inferior oblique, inferior rectus, superior rectus, *and* the left trochlear nucleus. The result, with short latency between nuclear discharge and muscle action involving the eyes: a corrective saccade involving the left inferior oblique and inferior rectus acting on the left eye, and an equal saccade of contralateral superior rectus and the superior oblique acting on the right eye.

An irksomely assiduous student now wants to know about gaze with longer latency. She or he asks insistently, peering at me with Andalusian *mirada fuerte*. I tell that student that the interstitial nucleus of Cajal is involved in *mirada fuerte* (probably not the rostral interstitial nucleus of the MLF), but, not to worry: what we should do right now is relax, stop, think. What we've reviewed is sufficient for our purpose. You have to control *both* eyes, right? And you have to do so adhering all the while to Ewald Hering's law of equal innervation involving eyes on either side of the midline.

Yoked muscles necessitate decussation. The MLF and the trochlear decussation are eminently apparent at gestational week ten.

7

After the Tenth Week

I have a friend and colleague who tried once, on a stratospherically ambitious whim, to teach neuroanatomy to twelve students . . . just using words. No photomicrographs, no Powerpoint presentations, not even the dissection of brains. His course occupied a two-month block in the curriculum, back in the days when true experiments in pedagogy were encouraged at my medical school. I'm all for that freedom and always will be, but, at the time, I thought he was nuts. He said that the exercise tasked him—and, more importantly, forced his students—to communicate what's important as lucidly as possible. In this monograph, I've adopted his odd but brilliant approach, especially in the next few pages.

Chapter before last, we left off at the tenth week of gestation. Commissures and decussations are just visible. In the lower brainstem, we have the medial longitudinal fasciculus and the trochlear decussation. Above and below the third ventricle, we have dorsal and ventral crossings. The posterior commissure is dorsal. The anterior commissure and the primordial corpus callosum are anterior and more ventral. The optic chiasm is most ventral. According to a mantra of brain development, we have CLOSED the cranial neuropore and DIVIDED into rudimentary cerebral hemispheres. Lower down, in the brainstem, we've also DIVIDED orthogonally to the long-axial midline into a basal (ventral) plate versus an alar (dorsal) plate; the demarcation between the two is the sulcus limitans of His.

Beginning no earlier than the eighth week, neurons PROLIFERATE. They do so well past the tenth week. Where do the neurons proliferate and where do they go?

*

In the midbrain at 5-10 gestational weeks, there's a tectum and a tegmentum that roughly correlate to the alar and basal plates, respectively. In the diencephalon at 5-10 weeks, we no longer have a basal plate at all; we only have an alar plate.

The diencephalon and structures rostral to it are *all* of alar origin. The diencephalic ventral alar plate will have (more or less) only motor nuclei, just as the basal plate is "motoric" in the brainstem and spinal cord. The diencephalic dorsal alar plate will have (more or less) only sensory nuclei, just as the alar plate is "sensory" in the brainstem and spinal cord.

In this developing diencephalon, the ventral alar part matures into hypothalamus, the dorsal alar part into thalamus (and more, as we'll see).

To conceptualize where neuroblasts, fated to become cortical neurons, proliferate, think about a most bizarre open-faced sandwich. It's a hollow sphere of bread covered by whatever you like on your bread— say, it's peanut butter. The hollow of the sphere is the third ventricle. The lower half of the spherical sandwich is ventral alar, destined to be hypothalamus; the upper half is dorsal alar, destined to be thalamus as well as cortex. Viewed from the outside, we see no bread in our structure. It looks like a sphere of peanut butter.

Now we apply anatomical terms to our sandwich. Bread equals a so-called "mantle layer."[1] Peanut butter equals a so-called "marginal layer." Early neurons pseudostratify in the mantle layer. The marginal

---

[1] "Mantle layer" in my analogy conflates so-called matrix and mantle layers. And I do not mention the innermost ependymal layer, again for the sake of simplicity.

layer contains pluripotent neuroepithelial cells, some of which will differentiate into glial cells.

Cells that mature into cortical neurons proliferate in the bread on the inside, not the peanut butter on the outside.

The hemispheres derive entirely from the dorsal half of our sandwich, *only* from the dorsal alar plate. Neocortical neurons originate in the dorsal mantle layer, but they migrate across the dorsal marginal layer to form bread on the outside.

The dorsal half of our open-faced sandwich with peanut butter on the outside metamorphoses into a proper sandwich consisting of two pieces of bread and peanut butter between the slices. Outside bread equals developing neocortex. Peanut butter equals white matter deep to neocortex. Inside bread equals the mantle layer.

The two-piece-of-bread sandwich is temporary. To steal a peek at the telos or endpoint, we'll eventually re-achieve an open-faced sandwich with bread on the outside and peanut butter on the inside.

*

The life clock now reads three months' gestation.

We have before us a curious, bilobed sandwich.

Radial migration across the dorsal marginal layer forms bread on the outside. Neuronal proliferation and radial migration are robust, so much so that the outer bread layer eventually folds upon itself in literal gyrations. The two hemispheres connect to each other by a growing corpus callosum, which had started as a primordium just anterior to the anterior commissure. By the fifteen week of gestation, the corpus callosum forms a roof over the third ventricle. More and more white-matter axons cross the midline to the other hemisphere.

Neurons travel radially to get from the mantle layer across the marginal layer to the surface, but not all deep-bread neurons migrate in that way. Grey matter structures like the thalamus, corpus striatum, claustrum, amygdala, and olfactory cortex take their origin in the dorsal mantle layer and their neurons remain deep to the dorsal marginal layer.

The dorsal mantle layer dissipates in time.

The neocortex (bread on the outside) forms up to six layers of neurons; the underlying peanut-butter layer thickens as white matter becomes increasingly abundant.

Another great task is underway as the second trimester proceeds, aside from development of neocortex just described. Tracts form. They differ from interhemispheric commissures in that they cross from one side of the body towards the brain on the contralateral side, not from one side of the brain to the other. These ascending, decussating sensory pathways appear before the first hints of a descending corticospinal tract in ontogeny.

8

"Fate"

When we read about an axonal fate either to cross or not to cross the midline, there's a tendency to refer to axons as if they possessed intelligence and indulged fastidious, personal preferences. For example, an axon "recognizes" the axial midline; it is "attracted" to it or "repelled" by it; if it crosses the midline, it does so like Caesar crossing his river Rubicon, fated never to return. My etymological dictionary tells me that "axon" has its root in the word "axis." Axons and axes relate to each other. I'm interested to understand some basics about axons and the body's midline, since commissures and decussations both traverse it. There's a great deal of literature that we might review. As has been obvious from the start, however, my goal hasn't been an encyclopedic review of anything. The original "why?" still buzzes in my head.

Does sensory information from my hand on one side get pulled somehow towards its destination in contralateral thalamus and somatosensory cortex, as if by tropism? Starting roughly in the ninth week of gestation, does a right brain start to push a pyramidal tract towards the left spinal cord? A mature axon–just to dispel any thought that I abused etymology a few sentences ago–has its own, often very, very long axis, hence the anatomical term "axon." But, in the development of pathways, axons start as nubbins. They lengthen under influences acting at growth cones at the tips of axons. When fibers arrive at the midline, we can read about their molecularly determined "fates." What determines the determinism?

An elegant study, published in 1983 (Lumsden and Davies), depicts phenomena that are anything but straightforward. In the mouse, the trigeminal ganglion appears on the ninth embryonic day (E9); by the tenth day (E10), roughly 1,200 axonal tendrils extend from the ganglion towards the maxilla of the murine face (five percent of the total at E13), but they don't reach the maxillary "whisker field" until the twelfth day (E12).

The authors' several experiments called for explants of ganglionic tissue from days E10 and E11 to be co-cultured with explants from the face and from an "inappropriate target," a forelimb bud. All explants were of the same embryonic age. Exquisitely created, little wells in culture dishes held the samples of tissue; the distance between explants in a dish was the distance between the trigeminal ganglion and the whisker field. Cultures incubated for 48 hours. The authors wondered where ganglionic tendrils (called neurites) would head and how they would travel to their destination.

A first experiment found: if ganglionic explant cultures just by itself with no other wells in the dish, no neurites form. The authors kept looking for 72 hours after the 48 hours of culture time.

A second experiment found: if the ganglionic well sits between a well containing forelimb bud and another containing face, neurites extend to the facial well directly. Divide the space around the ganglionic well into four parts: a quadrant facing the facial well, a quadrant facing the forelimb-bud well, then two others above and below. The neurites extend only to the first of the four quadrants, like a dead-straight, center-of-the-cup putt in golf. Neurites don't head to the forelimb bud well, period.

A third experiment found: if you set up three wells with facial extract to the far left, then two ganglionic wells next to each other in a line, then neurites from the further-away ganglionic well (further away from the facial well, only in the quadrant facing the facial well, despite the fact that the distance between the distant well and the face is now doubled) exceeds the number of neurites that form in the near ganglionic well in its quadrant facing away from the facial well. As long as you face the face, neurites head there.

A fourth experiment found: if you culture E12, not E10 or E11, ganglionic extract together with facial and forelimb wells, then neurites extend to the forelimb well—which is without precedent in this study. Neurites of the E12 extract that extend to the facial well do so like breaking putts entering from the top and bottom of the proverbial cup, but there are still neurites that straight putt to the facial well in the quadrant facing the face.

There's more to the paper, but we're in a position to consider its essentials.

In anatomy class, we're used to looking at a structure like the trigeminal ganglion, then we utter tediously, "this is the trigeminal ganglion." How does a person know? Well, it looks like the trigeminal ganglion. It's located in the right place, so what else could it be? Statements about "the right place" have much developmental neuroscience behind them, and it's not irrelevant to remind ourselves that, like an annelid worm, we're composed of metameric segments to start. Then, location along the anterior-posterior axis determines differential function. Another way of saying the same thing is: there's segment-specific identity. One could make the argument that segment-specific neurites heading to face make sense, because the rhombomere in question is not at the level of the forelimb. It's at the level of face. We avoid saying that the axon "knows" to go the whisker field, because it doesn't know any such thing. Segmental identity is like a plan already in place before any neurites appear in the first place.

The manner in which neurites head to their target is direct, by shortest apparent route, but travel differs depending on the day. The authors hypothesized some precisely timed chemotaxis along a concentration gradient between wells. The hypothesis still has legs today, as we'll discuss. The paper didn't identify a responsible chemical, but would a hypothetical "trigeminal neurotropic factor" explain what they observed? We've already delved a bit into many forces at play. Proper chemotaxis depends on the rhombomere. In the absence of appropriate target tissue, there are no neurites at all. If on the wrong day, we have errant neurites. Timing is also key.

In general, chemotaxis changes some random movement or growth into a particular direction; it's a reduction in disorder. But chemotaxis alone can't explain the fated destination of a neurite. There are other considerations, as a widening gyre of papers on guidance attests. To have a fate is quite complex biology.

Beware of the word "complex." Often it means, "we dunno."

*

If we think geometrically, an axis is a line without breadth that separates sides, top from bottom, front from back. A neural axis is different. It can be defined chemically as something with volume and content. In spinal cord preparations, diffusible proteins along the midline have been isolated; the first among them (related to crossings) were named netrins. I should be specific: netrin-1 concentrates at the cord's ventral surface along the longitudinal midline, with a concentration gradient ventral to dorsal (high to low concentration) along *that* bottom-to-top midline. What we mean by "midline" has already become more complicated than a line in geometry.

Netrin-1 interacts with axonal growth-cone receptors belonging to a receptor family deleted in colorectal cancer, hence "DCC." Netrin-1 occupying a DCC receptor guides axons to where netrin-1 is most concentrated—i.e., towards the midline. The Netrin-1-DCC interaction is a long-range molecular mechanism of axonal guidance, but there's debate about what defines "long range." We might be talking about just millimeters.

Getting to the midline is no promise that an axon will cross it. But let's say that an axon does cross; what's to prevent a netrin-DCC interaction to force a return to the midline? If there's a chemo-attractant mechanism, there must be a chemo-repellent one, right? Here's where things get complicated: netrins don't attract all axons to the midline (sometimes they repel axons from the midline); interactions between a different protein called Slit and growth-cone receptors belonging to a family called Roundabout (Robo) *also* repel axons from the midline.

Netrin-1 and Slit are by no means the only molecules hugging the midline ("semaphorins," "ephrins," and "Draxin" are also there, all of them "repulsive"); then, on top of it all, there are gradients of morphogens along the rostral-caudal axis.

We've encountered morphogens previously. Recall sonic hedgehog (the protein) and its role in morphogenesis. We discussed SHH gene mutations in association with holoprosencephaly in chapter five. Along the rostral-caudal axis, the midline concentration of sonic hedgehog varies from low (rostrally) to high (caudally). The longitudinal gradient, in addition to the ventral-dorsal gradient at any one level, influences axonal attraction to or repulsion from the midline. Adding to the mix: how morphogens influence axonal direction depends on whether the axon is precommissural or postcommissural.

To me, the most important thought regarding axonal guidance has to do with the verb "to depend." We learned from the seminal 1983 study that E10 and E11 neurites move a certain way; E12 neurites a different, less elegant way. What happens depends on timing.

Netrin-1 interacts with DCC, we said. Well, it depends: repellent Draxin also interacts with DCC.

Netrin-1-DCC operates in counterpoint to Slit-Robo, we might infer as a generalization. Well, it depends: if an axon hasn't crossed the midline, the Slit gradient at the midline doesn't seem to matter at all, but if an axon has crossed, then the Netrin midline gradient doesn't seem to matter at all. Much depends on when receptors and which receptors are expressed at the axonal tip.

If we know about Netrin-1-DCC and Slit-Robo, at least we have the basics, could we not say? Well, it depends: where you happen to be along the neuraxis (rostral? caudal?) also matters, and different locations invoke differing gradients of morphogens.

Good news, there are take-home points:

1. "Fate" is a vague term compared to a statement such as "Netrin-1-DCC interaction facilitates guidance to the midline." But the

statement doesn't say anything about the why of decussation. On the other hand, perhaps there is a well-wrought destiny that we have both crossed *and* uncrossed pathways.
2. The axes of the neuraxis are busy places, not lines of simple division. The "contents" of the midline(s) have much to do with control of axonal movement and direction. Why would there be so many mechanisms of control if the difference between crossing and not crossing were unimportant?
3. How axons reach their destinations depends not only on local factors at any given axial level, but also on their points of origin along the longitudinal neuraxis, since rostral-caudal gradients are in play as well.

9

A Note about Cartography

There are anatomists who go to the trouble for us to display the brain as if it existed in only two dimensions. The value of such a map has to do with organizing neuroanatomy and even developmental neuroanatomy in a Cartesian-coordinate way.

Let's use the Earth in a Mercator projection as an example of a flat map. Latitudes of the globe are all the same length as the equator; longitudes are also of the same length. More importantly, latitudes and longitudes are at exact, right angles to each other. A random line on the map (called a rhumb) can indicate true direction without need to account for the earth's curvature. The Mercator projection distorts sizes of land masses, but a flat map proves useful when plotting a course, say, at sea.

If one had such a map of the neuraxis, we could figure out starting points and termini by x and y coordinates only. If I were a pyramidal cell axon departing the arm portion of the primary motor homunculus, then I'd start at some x,y place, then move to some other, specific x,y coordinate (I'd maintain a position relative to an axon from leg domain of the homunculus), then follow my rhumb lines all the way to my destination in the ventral spinal cord. For any given quadrant and segment of travel, it might be possible to discover the morphogen or other chemical gradients in two dimensions governing my route.

In preparing for this chapter and the last one, it was hard not to obsess over a sentence from Lumsden and Krumlauf (1996): "Patterning of cell types [in the vertebrate neuraxis] appears to be organized on a Cartesian grid of positional information, the coordinates of which correspond with the AP [anterior-posterior] and dorsoventral (DV) axes of the neural tube: analyses of cell fate after experimental rotation of the neural plate have indicated that regional fate is determined along the AP axis before and independently of fate restriction on the DV axis." If a cell's fate in the nervous system (to become a motor neuron or something else) can be determined by location, why can't an axon's route of travel also be so determined, since we know that morphogens also influence an axon's rhumb-line directions?

Recall a couple of statements from the last chapter. Here they are, cut and pasted: ". . . it's not irrelevant to remind ourselves that, like an annelid worm, we're composed of metameric segments to start. Then, location along the anterior-posterior axis determines differential function." At that time, I tried to characterize segment-specific identity in the spirit of Lumsden and Krumlauf. Presently, I plead guilty to redundant syntax that may have annoyed the medical student to the point of distraction.

My dictionary says that a metamere is "one in a series of homologous body segments, as in worms and lobsters." A metamere *is* a segment, so "metameric segments" repeats itself. Here's a proponent of 2D brain maps (Swanson, 2012) talking about why segmentation matters in biology: "The basic idea is that this arrangement [segmentation] is a genetically efficient way to program the development of a more complex animal because essentially the same genetic program can be used over and over–in each segment or metamere." Next, I'll quote him along with his coauthors from 1995; he says much the same thing, but with specific reference to somites of the body: "One established way to reduce the total number of genes required for morphogenesis is the use of segments or metameres: serially repeating units such as somites that share a primary morphological plan and underlying genetic program, although each segment may go on to form distinguishing secondary features." He's not talking about brain metameres (neuromeres) or genetic metamerism (repetitive expression of genes in different neuromeres), though one thinks that he would have loved, in the 1990's, to have proven both. We'll turn to the subject of neuromeres in a moment.

Swanson's work should interest us because of an idea implicit in using any 2D brain map, especially one that has like segments/quadrants in it: to find a way, you repeat redirections along rhumbs, quadrant by quadrant, as if in a Mercator projection. In the case of the pyramidal tract, the redirections would *eventually* point to a specific destination in the body far away, but not at the start of travel. A left-frontal axonal growth cone might position itself relative to some vector pointing caudally (it might head just "south" based on local genetic, epigenetic, or chemical cues), only later to be directed, nudged, towards the spinal cord, after many, many intricate redirections, including the one across the midline at the cervicomedullary junction, roughly where the head transitions to the rest of the body.

*

On the subject of 2D maps, I'd be remiss not to mention Nieuwenhuys (2011). Influenced by the work of C. Judson Herrick in the early 20th century and of Wilhelm His (Senior) in the 19th, among others, he flattened the brainstem in maps of many kinds of fish.

The medical student protests, "oh, why fish, why now?" Answer: because we get to review some material.

In flattened fish brainstems, all that we learned in our chapters five and seven—about basal and alar plates in the medulla and spinal cord; tectum (alar-like) and tegmentum (basal-like) in midbrain; dorsal and ventral alar plates in the diencephalon; the alar origin of diencephalon and all other structures rostral to it, including the dorsal alar origin of the hemispheres–, absolutely all of that, returns with a vengeance along with an observation that might escape notice in 3D.

Looking at the brainstem in any routine transverse, sagittal, or coronal section, you wouldn't immediately surmise that medulla, pons, and midbrain altogether organize into vertical columns. But if you flatten, for example, the midbrain into two dimensions, then dorsal, tectal structures appear lateral to the tegmentum. Those midbrain tectal structures, now displaced into a 2D map of the whole brainstem, look contiguous with vertical columns that pass below, through, and above the midbrain. Moreover, the columns (four of them) can be divided into more than a dozen segments (neuromeres) from hindbrain to cortex itself, Nieuwenhuys says. Neuromeres stack on top of each other like quadrants along a north-south longitude.

There are implications of his claim—at least, questions—that might change how we think about neural development. Is the cortex (and thalamus, hypothalamus, all of the brainstem, and, of course, the spinal cord) constructed from repetitive segments? Could the basic plan be that straightforward? Do subsets of segments destined to become cortex, thalamus, etc. really evince genetic metamerism? You could argue that all the above is artifact or artifice: you've squashed a 3D thing; naturally it looks different as a result. Does the changed look justify a rethinking of brain morphogenesis?

Maybe.

Or we might just observe that there's practicality in an organized, Cartesian coordinate system, as 2D maps of the brain and the world illustrate.

10

Point A to . . . ?

We've either alluded to or traced the following commissures and decussating tracts:
- pyramidal/corticospinal tract,
- lemniscal pathway,
- anterolateral system,
- tectospinal tract,
- rubrospinal tract,
- decussation of the superior cerebellar peduncles,
- optic chiasm,
- posterior commissure,
- habenular commissure,
- corpus callosum,
- hippocampal commissure,
- anterior commissure,
- medial longitudinal fasciculus,
- and the trochlear decussation.

Aside from the fact that midline crossing happens in all instances, is there another common feature? Maybe what I have to say next isn't perfect, but I think it's worth noticing that if you travel any of the above paths, you depart towards some destination that reflects, mirrors, or even reduplicates your point of origin.

In chapter three, we talked about the body's three dimensions and brain maps of the body. Here I focus on how a crossing path gets us from one brain place (point A) to a homologous place or places elsewhere in the brain. You could call the destination a discrete "point B"–true enough, point B exists physically elsewhere in the brain. But it's a kind of "point A 'prime,'" a place/places that could remind you from whence you came, even if you've navigated quadrants away.

Consider the corpus callosum. From its genu to splenium, fibers pass from one hemisphere to the other such that there's a connection from one prefrontal area to the contralateral prefrontal area (at the genu); then one primary motor area to the other (about midway in the body of the corpus callosum); then one primary somatosensory area to the other a bit further back. At the splenium, one primary visual area connects to the other. One appreciates why R.W. Sperry (1961) refers to hemispheric nodes of connection as "mirror mates."

In microelectrode recordings described by Hubel (1995), stimuli presented to both eyes in the vertical midline elicited responses from visual fibers of the splenium, suggesting an interhemispheric crosstalk or overlap between hemispheric representations of visual space. The receptive fields for splenial responses cluster at the visual midline, whether an animal looks up, down, or gazed straight ahead. Hubel referred to those fibers as "cement" between halves of the visual world. Seeing in front of your nose, as I tried to explore anatomically in chapter four, is bihemispheric. Prerequisite for the task (I tried to thread needle, if you recall) are crossed *and* uncrossed connections. The optic chiasm is a premier example of partial decussation, with its crossed and uncrossed connections to visual cortex.

Though more involved in terms of anatomy, we can think about the superior cerebellar peduncle as a decussation from one homunculus to other, homologous ones. Elsewhere, we've mentioned homunculi in the neuraxis (think about three of them lined up next to each other at Brodman's areas 3a, 3b, 1, and 2). The finer the resolution of our anatomy, the more we see how wiring and decussation organize some or many plots of the body, of space, or of both. To repeat myself, the plots are homologous, not quite "mirror mates," but fundamentally related to each other nevertheless.

Axons that contribute to the superior cerebellar peduncle arise in the dentate nucleus, the most lateral of the deep cerebellar nuclei. The dentate nucleus is a structure best seen, perhaps only seen, in mammals, and it is particularly developed (it's large) in apes and humans. Its alleged resemblance to teeth mystifies me; or, one could say it's dental but horribly in need of orthodontia. On either side of the pontine rostral-caudal midline, nestled in the white matter of the middle cerebellar peduncle, in axial section they look to me like two very winding rivers that form the rough shape of parentheses whose concavities face each other.

The rostral dentate on either side projects, via a decussating superior cerebellar peduncle, to a part of the contralateral red nucleus (parvocellular, with small cells, but the largest area of that nucleus in humans) and also to ventrolateral thalamic nuclei which in turn project somatotopically to motor cortices. Note the plural; we're not talking about just the primary motor cortex.

The caudal dentate on either side projects, via a decussating superior cerebellar peduncle, to contralateral, parvocellular red nucleus; to other places we won't discuss, including contralateral superior colliculus; and to ventro- and dorso-medial thalamic nuclei which in turn project to this astonishing list of places, located all over the contralateral hemisphere (Nieuwenhuys, 2008):

prefrontal cortex,

frontal and supplementary eye fields,

medial intraparietal and rostral inferior parietal areas.

Anatomist Brodal (1981) teaches me that if you electrically stimulate in the dentate, you can record responses in specific areas of motor cortex, depending on where you stimulated in the dentate. You can even elicit contractions in the limbs with such cerebellar nuclear stimulation. Both observations corroborate that there's somatotopy in the dentate nucleus. But there's more to the cerebellothalamocortical projection than a repetition of homunculi. Brodal writes in his textbook, "These and other observations suggest that there must be a topological organization throughout the entire cerebellothalamocortical projection. This does not necessarily mean that there is a point-to-point arrangement throughout this route."

The question posed in my chapter's title could be edited: "Is There No Point-to-Point?" For some teachers and students in medical school, news that "no, there isn't" might evoke a child's disappointment when told the truth about Santa Claus. Most children, though, have already guessed as much by the time we tell them.

*

If you examine small areas of the dentate in tracer studies, dentate nuclear to thalamic nuclear connections seem precise. Entire somatotopic representations in dentate and ventral thalamic nuclei match each other as homologues. Stimulating a spot in the dentate results in a short-latency activation of a restricted area in a thalamic nucleus, as one expects. But then there's a long-latency activation of a much larger area in that thalamic nucleus. Why the latter?

Downstream in the cerebellothalamocortical projection, you can stimulate multiple, widely spaced areas in ventrolateral nucleus of thalamus only to elicit a cortical response from a small, discrete area of cortex. Or you can stimulate in the dentate, upstream in the projection, to activate a rather large area of cortex. We already know that thalamocortical projections ramify–"spew" might be a better verb– across swaths of cortex.

Brodal, whose evidence I'm rehearsing, forewarned us not to assume point-to-point correlations. Original point A doesn't lead neatly to a point B, to the consternation of those who just want to know how axons get from place to place. Notice, however, that all along the cerebellothalamocortical projection, there are homologues of the body: in dentate nucleus, ventrolateral thalamic nucleus, and even in diverse cortical locales. All are connected to each other in the projection we've been discussing.

It's commonly said that for every forty afferents entering cerebellum, there's only one efferent fiber. Much, though not all, of the input to one hemisphere of cerebellum comes from the homolateral side of the body. 40x "in" reduces to 1x "out", but the downstream effect of 1x can be either exquisitely focal or of grander, wider scale. A lot depends on how different somatotopies, all homologues of each other, interact—not only in the cerebellothalamocortical projection.

*

I've always wondered why there are so many somatotopic representations throughout the brain. Take just the ventral thalamic nuclei as an example: each of them possesses somatotopic organization, both in motor and sensory nuclei in that ventral nuclear tier. All homunculi refer to the same body, right? Why are there so many of representations of the same body—and, in what way, precisely, do they "interact"?

I think it would be absurd and wrong to say that we know "how." But we know enough not to conclude something that's probably flat wrong—for example, that there's no neural processing that happens between nodes—homuncular representations—in any given projection.

There's a famous analogy that comes to mind, though, honestly, it has nothing to do with homunculi. I'll use it nevertheless, for fun, and mainly because it helps me think.

Imagine that there's windowless room full of clocks and assorted timepieces; all of them work and they all tell time. There are big ones and small ones, a couple of pendulum clocks and few digital ones among them. A person without a watch walks into the room interested to know what time it is. It would appear that she has arrived at a good place for information. She picks up the first timepiece she sees. It says noon or midnight. She's curious to know whether all the clocks tell the same time, and she's understandably curious to find one of those 24-hour clocks to learn the true time of day, noon or midnight. In the absence of light from any window, she has no idea of day or night. She starts to check all the clocks.

You're curious to know whether it was noon or midnight. But that particular information is not quite the point.

In the famous version of the analogy, used in philosophy courses, it turns out all the clocks tell the same time. But you can't say–it's illogical to maintain–that one timepiece influences the other. You might think there's mutual influence (because why would they all being telling the same time?), but you can't prove it.

I'm interested only in three things: 1. She enters the room; 2. She checks; 3. She leaves.

I'll risk generalizations based on my analogy, though I still have the cerebellothalamocortical projection primarily in mind. There's input into a room. Multiple nodes (all homologous, like so many timepieces) exist in that room. There's output from the room.

We have no idea about noon versus midnight.

Her entry, checking, and departure are subjects for our next, second-to-last chapter.

*

Before we leave this one, however, I'll discuss a case (Yachnis and Rorke, 1999) for the purpose of talking about the dysgenesis of decussations.

We don't know a lot about the adult life or family history of a 31 year-old man who came to autopsy. He had been found submerged in a swimming pool.

We have more information about his infancy and childhood. There was developmental delay: he walked at 42 months, about 30 months late; he started to combine words at 5 years, the approximate age when American children enter kindergarten. He had a congenital nystagmus. We don't have further details about the nystagmus.

At some point, he developed an oculomotor apraxia. I wonder whether the apraxia was congenital, not acquired, but all the same I visualize that he can't generate a saccade, say, to the left. He thrusts his head to the left to fix the eyes on the target. There's an issue: short-latency correction happens normally with a head thrust (when head thrusts left, eyes turn conjugately to the right to maintain objects on the foveae). But he wants to look left. So the head movement overshoots the mark (to the far left), then he adjusts his head just a bit to the right, to accomplish a new fixation on the left target. Horizontal saccades in either direction are impaired in congenital oculomotor apraxias, often with preserved vertical eye movements.

As a kid, he stuck his tongue out of his mouth a lot. A partial cleft palate had been noted at birth. At one year of age, he developed seizures which apparently continued through his life. But at the time of his death three decades later, he had been seizure free for six years.

His gait, we're told, had "always" been wide based and ataxic.

And that's all we know in terms of history and physical examination.

The original report of the syndrome in question (Joubert et al., 1969) tells the story of four affected children in one French-Canadian family. The authors traced the family tree back 11 generations to learn that consanguineous marriages happened in the 17th century and perhaps in the 19th.

Our 31 year-old gentleman's story doesn't much resemble any of the original four cases, save for many suggestions of ataxia and incoordination, nystagmus, and various eye movement abnormalities (but there's no obvious oculomotor apraxia in the original four cases). The 1969 report emphasized episodic hyperpnea, which was not a feature of our man's history. Reports in the last decade or so underscore the phenotypic variability of Joubert syndrome. Two genetic linkages are now known, to chromosomes nine and eleven.

The interest in our case is the neuropathology. Here are the highlights:

a smallish brain (1,340 grams) with a "simple gyral pattern," but six-layered neocortex in both hemispheres, with grossly normal basal ganglia;

presence of a corpus callosum;

aplasia of the cerebellar vermis, a key feature in all cases reported in 1969;

loss of Purkinje cells in cerebellum;

fragmented dentate nuclei;

abnormal decussation of the superior cerebellar peduncles, with marked elongation of the rostral extent of the fourth ventricle;

loss of reticular formation neurons;

anomalies of dorsal column nuclei (also, fasciculi gracilis and cuneatus were not distinct tracts);

complete absence of the pyramidal decussation;

and other findings.

I'm genuinely curious how he made it to 31 years.

A study of five, phenotypically various pedigrees (Ferland et al., 2004) gives us reason to believe that profound developmental delay, mental retardation, and autism characterize the lives of those afflicted by Joubert syndrome.

Given the above constellation of abnormalities at autopsy, the authors of our case report hypothesized an onset of deformations before the tenth gestational week, perhaps at six-to-eight weeks–i.e., at a time of active neuronal proliferation. At post-mortem, the corpus callosum was present, so defect onset couldn't have happened after the tenth week.

The maturation of decussations and an individual's progress towards a more fully functional brain seem coincident.

11

The Room

In clinical work, we feel an urge to localize. It's a hunger of mind, like the insatiable curiosity to learn "what the MRI says." (Let's be honest. We're routinely eager to see the imaging, because we like looking at brains.) One clue that neurology, neurosurgery, or neuropathology is in your future is a capacity just to stare at the anatomy–radiographic or real–for hours on end. And I do mean hours. Before you are even cognizant of time's passing, hours become years, then decades. But the brain isn't composed of excellent localizations. Parcellate it if you like, smash it flat, bisect it, or vivsect what otherwise keeps it together, but it's a whole thing. It's a single, cavernous room packed with information.

Chapter ten's analogy isn't about an unvisited room. My interest has to do with comings and goings in and out; the processes inside the room aren't fully known, though contemporary neuroscientists, like the woman without a watch, never cease to investigate the contents.

We're about to revisit the great decussating pathway called the corticospinal/pyramidal tract, which we first sketched at the start of this monograph. We've since learned that crossing the midline is highly regulated, whether we're discussing a commissure or a decussation. We know that crossings exist, some just as primordia, as early as the tenth week of gestation. The corpus callosum is seen that early, but better examples happen even earlier and more caudally, like the medial longitudinal fasciculus.

You can survive into adult life without a pyramidal decussation, as we saw in the case of Joubert's syndrome. Presumably, uncrossed motor fibers can take control of the body's sides. Other anomalies in that case—the disarray of the gracile and cuneate fasciculi, the fragmentation of Purkinje cell layer in cerebellum and of the output dentate nucleus, and the dysgenesis of the decussation of the superior cerebellar peduncles—lead to the surmise that some prominent decussations, including the pyramidal decussation, must transpire in normal development after the tenth week of gestation. We know as much because certain words reverberate in the ear: "a given brain malformation may not have its onset after a developmental event is completed." What happens after CLOSURE and DIVISION? PROLIFERATION. Abnormalities of decussation could relate to errant neuronal proliferation.

Let's now add a statement from Sarnat and Netsky (2002), that at no stage in brain development do primary sensory and motor neurons constitute a majority of all neurons. From the very start of neuronal differentiation (recall our spherical sandwich from chapter seven), internuncial neurons or interneurons always predominate, Sarnat and Netsky say.

In major sensory systems like the lemniscal pathway and spinothalamic tract, second-order neurons (by definition, they are interneurons) traverse the midline. The medical student is quick to notice that the long, pyramidal cell axon arising in a fifth layer somewhere in frontal cortex doesn't synapse with a second-order neuron. That axon itself crosses the midline at the pyramidal decussation at the cervicomedullary junction. On the ventral surface of the low medulla we can see with our own eyes how the decussation effaces the anterior median fissure.

We've discussed much of the above already, although Sarnat and Netsky offer a new fact that's probably true. Surely, there's no more to say.

There's just the tawdry matter of entering and leaving "the room." The medical student opines: "sensory input, motor output; it's basic biology. The room is the brain; I get it."

Let's step for a moment beyond basics.

A hegemony of interneurons causes me to rethink what the corticospinal tract is. There's no better example, one would think, of a motor neuron than a fifth-layer Betz cell and its long axon. But what if the corticospinal tract is internuncial (literally, a "go-between") itself? Read Davidoff's spin on the subject (1990): ". . . we can regard the PT [pyramidal tract] as an internuncial pathway intercalated between subcortical structures (e.g., basal ganglia, cerebellum), cortical areas (e.g., premotor cortex, association cortex), and afferent inputs from peripheral sensory receptors and spinal motoneurons. As such, it occupies a central position as the site of convergence for several dispersed sets or neurons . . ."

Maybe crossed pathways are inside the room.

The go-between that shuttles between subcortex, premotor and sensory cortices and spinal cord—the decussating corticospinal tract—lives in the room. The pyramidal tract is internuncial in one other regard. Like the major decussating sensory pathways, it's a shuttle between hemibody and hemisphere.

What about the go-between that shuttles between cerebellar maps to cortical ones (decussation of the superior cerebellar peduncles)? Also inside.

The go-between that shuttles between retinal maps and visual cortical maps (optic chiasm)? See inside.

The go-between that shuttles mirror-mate locales of cortex (corpus callosum)? Ditto. We can stop with those examples.

Unfortunately, my room analogy explodes before my eyes. Inputs and outputs to the room depend on the crossing that we discuss. The contents of the room include all things internuncial, like decussations, commissures, probably also reentrant paths or closed circuits or wiring that we haven't begun to fathom either in our philosophy or neuroscience. The woman who just wanted to know the time goes away. We never learn whether it's noon or midnight.

The analogy has served its purpose, however. I may not have determined the telos of decussation, but I've placed crossing, like a large capital letter X, at the center of my neuroanatomical view.

12

Why?

Dunno exactly.
But I looked up a few items for you.
It's your turn to think about your answer.

REFERENCES

General Neuroanatomy:

Brodal A. *Neurological Anatomy in Relation to Clinical Medicine.* Third ed. New York/Oxford: Oxford University Press, 1981.

Carpenter MB, Sutin J. *Human Neuroanatomy.* Eighth ed. Baltimore/London: Williams and Wilkins, 1983.

Nieuwenhuys R, Voogd J, van Huijzen C. *The Human Central Nervous System.* Fourth ed. Berlin/Heidelberg/New York: Springer Verlag, 2008.

*

Other Books:

Hebb DO. *Essay on Mind.* New York: Psychology Press, 2009.

Hubel DH. *Eye, Brain, and Vision.* New York: Scientific American Library, 1995.

Langman J. *Medical Embryology.* Fourth ed. Baltimore: Williams and Wilkins, 1981.

Newton, I. *Opticks or A Treatise of the Reflections, Refractions, Inflections, & Colours of Light* [based on the fourth edition, London 1730]. New York: Dover, 1979.

Swanson LW. *Brain Architecture. Understanding the Basic Plan.* Second ed. New York: Oxford University Press, 2012.

Volpe JJ. *Neurology of the Newborn.* Second ed. Philadelphia: W.B. Saunders, 1987.

*

Articles:

Alvarez-Bolado G, Rosenfeld MG, Swanson LW. Model of forebrain regionalization based on spatiotemporal patterns of POU-III homeobox gene expression, birthdates, and morphological features. *Journal of Comparative Neurology* 1995;355:237-295.

Anonymous. Cerebral localisation. *British Medical Journal* 1877;2:699.

Bender M. Brain control of conjugate horizontal and vertical eye movements. A survey of the structural and functional correlates. *Brain* 1980:103;23-69.

Chisholm A, Tessier-Lavigne M. Conservation and divergence of axon guidance mechanisms. *Current Opinion in Neurobiology* 1999;9:603-615.

Collett T. Stereopsis in toads. *Nature* 1977;267:349-351.

Crelin ES, Netter FH, Shapter RK. Development of the nervous system. A logical approach to neuroanatomy. *Clinical Symposia* 1974;26(2), reprinted as a monograph, Summit, NJ: Ciba-Geigy, 1974.

Davidoff RA. The pyramidal tract. *Neurology* 1990;40:332-339.

De Lussanet MHE, Osse JWM. An ancestral twist explains the contralateral forebrain and the optic chiasm in vertebrates. *Animal Biology* 2012;62:193-216.

Dickson BJ. Molecular mechanisms of axon guidance. *Science* 2002;298:1959-1964.

Dickson BJ, Zou Y. Navigating intermediate targets: the nervous system midline. *Cold Spring Harbor Perspectives in Biology* 2010;2:a002055.

Echelard Y, Epstein DJ, St-Jacques B, Shen L, Mohler J, McMahon JA, McMahon AP. Sonic hedgehog, a member of a family of putative signaling molecules, is implicated in the regulation of CNS polarity. *Cell* 1993;75:1417-1430.

Ferland RJ, Eyaid W, Collura RV, Tully LD, Hill RS, Al-Nouri D, Al-Rumayyan A, Topcu M, Gascon G, Bodell A, Shugart YY, Ruvolo M, Walsh CA. Abnormal cerebellar development and axonal decussation due to mutations in *AHI1* in Joubert syndrome. *Nature Genetics* 2004;36:1008-1013.

Florence SL, Wall JT, Kaas JH. Somatotopic organization of inputs from the hand to the spinal gray and cuneate nucleus of monkeys with observations on the cuneate nucleus of humans. *Journal of Comparative Neurology* 1989;286:48-70.

Gilles FH. Myelination in the neonatal brain. *Human Pathology* 1976;7:244-248.

Hikosaka O. The habenula: from stress evasion to value-based decision-making. *Nature Reviews/Neuroscience* 2010;11:503-513.

Horn AKE, Leigh RJ. The anatomy and physiology of the ocular motor system. *Handbook of Clinical Neurology, Neuro-ophthalmology* (Third Series) 2011;102:21-69.

Jeffery G. Architecture of the optic chiasm and the mechanisms that sculpt its development. *Physiological Reviews* 2001;81:1393-1414.

Joubert M, Eisenring JJ, Robb JP, Andermann F. Familial agenesis of the cerebellar vermis. A syndrome of episodic hyperpnea, abnormal eye movements, and retardation. *Neurology* 1969;19:813-825.

Kinsbourne M. Somatic twist: a model for the evolution of decussation. *Neuropsychology* 2013;27:511-515.

Lumsden AGS, Davies AM. Earliest sensory nerve fibres are guided to peripheral targets by attractants other than nerve growth factor. *Nature* 1983;306:786-788.

Lumsden A, Krumlauf R. Patterning the vertebrate neuraxis. *Science* 1996;274:1109-1115.

Mueller F, O'Rahilly R. The first appearance of the future cerebral hemispheres in the human embryo at stage 14. *Anatomy and Embryology* 1988;177:495-511.

Nanni L, Ming JE, Bocian M, Steinhaus K, Bianchi DW, de Die-Smulders C, Giannotti A, Imaizumi K, Jones KL, Del Campo M, Martin RA, Meinecke P, Pierpont MEM, Robin NH, Young ID, Roessler E, Muenke M. The mutational spectrum of the Sonic Hedgehog gene in holoprosencephaly: SHH mutations cause a significant proportion of autosomal dominant holoprosencephaly. *Human Molecular Genetics* 1999;8:2479-2488.

Nieuwenhuys R. The structural, functional, and molecular organization of the brainstem. *Frontiers in Neuroanatomy* 2011;5:33. doi: 10.3389/fnana.2011.00033.

Sarnat HB, Netsky MG. When does a ganglion become a brain? Evolutionary origin of the central nervous system. *Seminars in Pediatric Neurology* 2002;9:240-253.

Shinbrot T, Young W. Why decussate? Topological constraints on 3D wiring. *The Anatomical Record* 2008;291:1278-1292.

Sperry RW. Cerebral organization and behavior. *Science* 1961;133:1749-1757.

Stoeckli ET. Understand axon guidance: are we nearly there yet? *Development* 2018;145, dev 151415, doi:10.1242/dev.151415.

Vulliemoz S, Raineteau O, Jabaudon D. Reaching beyond the midline: why are human brains cross wired? *Lancet Neurology* 2005;4:87-99.

Wadsworth WG, Hedgecock EM. Hierarchical guidance cues in the developing nervous system of C. elegans. *BioEssays* 1996;18:355-362.

Yachnis AT, Rorke LB. Neuropathology of Joubert syndrome. *Journal of Child Neurology* 1999;14:655-659.

www.ingramcontent.com/pod-product-compliance
Lightning Source LLC
Chambersburg PA
CBHW031544210526
45464CB00003B/1149